The EKG Pocket Survival Guide

Thomas Masterson, M.D., M.S.
Jonathan Handler, M.D.
Scott Tenner, M.D., M.P.H.
Todd Rothenhaus, M.D.

Residents, Departments of Health Care Sciences
and Emergency Medicine
The George Washington University
Washington, D.C.

Note: This text is designed as a educational supplement.
EKG analysis is performed by resposible clinicians who
do so in the setting of their full clinical judgement.

Trade name used in this book are the property of their
manufacturers.

Fourth Printing

the EKG Pocket Survival Guide
Copyright 1993 (c) International Medical Publishing, Inc.
International Medical Publishing, Inc.
Alexandria, Virginia.
ISBN 0-9634063-8-8

Introduction

This book is a pocket sized reminder of what you already know. While not encyclopedic, it offers examples of principle electrocardiographic patterns with associated basic criteria.

If you are just starting out, Dubin's **Rapid Interpretation of EKGs** is required reading. For more seasoned readers we recommend Marriot's **Practical Electrocardiography**.

Cardiovascular diagnosis is a synthesis of the history, physical, EKG, chest radiograph and laboratory evaluation. Many new clinicians dislike EKGs because they can be ambiguous and difficult to interpret.

Remember:

    1. Be systematic.

    2. Always compare the current tracing with previous tracings.

    3. A normal EKG does not rule out the possibility of serious cardiac disease (including acute MI).

We wish to thank Dr. Benjamin Dickens for his technical expertise in scanning EKGs. Thanks also goes to Drs. Martha Pierce and Alan Wasserman for their insights and editorial assistance.

Good luck.

The Authors

How to do an EKG

Today's EKG machines are sophisticated devices that theoretically make recording an EKG simple and precise. Become familiar with the use of any machine that you may be called upon to use in an urgent situation.

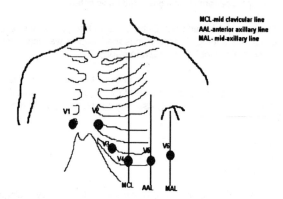

MCL-mid clavicular line
AAL-anterior axillary line
MAL- mid-axillary line

Lead Placement:

Limb leads are usually labeled but are also occasionally color coded so that:

Right arm- "White is on the right."
Right leg- "Green is for go" (Right leg is gas pedal).
Left leg- "Red is for stop" (Some brake with left leg).
Left arm- black lead.

Precordial leads are as follows: remember to palpate sternal angle adjacent to second rib and count downward.

V1- 4th intercostal space, right sternal border.
V2- 4th intercostal space, left sternal border.
V3- Between V2 and V4.
V4- Fifth intercostal space left mid clavicular line.
V5- Anterior axillary line at same level as V4.
V6- Mid axillary line at same level as V4.

Contents

Basic Cardiac Anatomy and Physiology

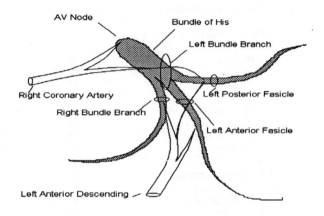

The Conducting System

The conducting system of the heart consists of the AV node, bundle of His, bundle branches and Purkinje system. The AV node is the only connection between the atria and ventricles except in Wolf-Parkinson-White(WPW) and Lown-Ganong-Levine (LGL) syndromes where tracts that bypass the AV node exist.

Basic Cardiac Anatomy and Physiology

Basic Cardiac Electrophysiology

The sinoatrial node (SA) initiates the sinus beat. Depolarization spreads out over the atria forming the P wave. Excitation slows at the AV node forming the PR segment. The stimulus travels down the His Bundle to the bundle branches and Purkinje system. The QRS represents the depolarization of the ventricles, while the T wave represents repolarization of the ventricles.

The Coronary Circulation

The right coronary artery (RCA) supplies the SA node, most AV nodes, the right atria, the right ventricle, the right bundle branch and occasionally the left posterior fascicle. The RCA divides to form the posterior descending artery (PDA) and a posterolateral branch. The right coronary may supply part of the apex and may anastomose with the left coronary.

The left coronary artery (LCA) consists of a short left main coronary artery which divides into the LCA anterior descending (LAD) and circumflex (Cx). The left supplies a minority of AV nodes, the left anterior fascicle and most left posterior fascicles. Branches of the LAD are called septal perforators. Branches of the circumflex are called obtuse marginals (OM). A large marginal is sometimes given off at the bifurcation of the LAD and circumflex and is known as a ramus intermedius.

EKG summary

1. Read name, date, and time on EKG.

2. Get old EKG for comparison.

3. Systematic evaluation:
   Rate
   Rhythm
   Axis -30° to +120° (variations in this normal range exist)
   Intervals
       PR < 0.21 and > 0.12 seconds
       QRS < 0.12 seconds
       QT interval
   Then PQRST...
       P wave morphology.
       Q waves.
       R wave progression.
       ST segments.
       T waves.
       U waves.

4. Interpretation: Arrhythmias, Hypertrophy, Blocks, Ischemia, Infarction, Metabolic effects, Drug effects.

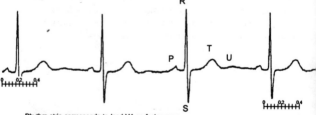

Rhythm strip corresponds to lead V4 on facing page.
Rate - 60 beats per minute.
Rhythm - sinus.
Intervals - PR = 0.14 seconds, QRS = 0.09 seconds, QT = 0.44 seconds.
Axis - leads I + and aVF +, axis is >0° and <90°, isoelectric between III and aVF, axis = 15°.
Normal P waves. No Q waves, normal R wave progression.
Normal ST segments. Upright T waves. Small U wave.
Interpretation: normal EKG.

2

Normal EKG

Name and date

While checking the name and date does not sound terribly sexy, it is the first step of interpreting a tracing. Without fail, the EKG you are handed or the EKG in the chart will someday belong to a patient other than the one you are evaluating. Obviously, sophisticated EKG reading skills are pointless if you are looking at the wrong tracing.

Once you know the name and date are correct, fold over the computer interpretation and do your own review of the tracing. Use the computer as a partner in teaching rather than a substitute for thinking.

Old EKG for comparison

Is it LVH with strain or lateral ischemia?
Are those Q waves new?
Only the old EKG will tell.

In the age of fax, every cardiac patient deserves the benefit of a comparison EKG.

Sources: 1. Old hospital chart.
              2. Primary physician.
              3. Outside hospital charts.
              4. EKG computer.

Inpatient EKGs should be compared with tracings from previous days.

Rate

By convention, EKG paper moves at 25 mm per second. The paper has big lines every 5 mm and little boxes every 1 mm. This produces the following relationships.

Each little box = 0.04 seconds.
Each big box = 0.20 seconds.

If the rate is regular and the distance between two QRS complexes is one big box, the rate is 300 beats per minute (bpm). Accordingly:

1 beat per big box equals	300 bpm.
2 boxes	150 bpm.
3 boxes	100 bpm.
4 boxes	75 bpm.
5 boxes	60 bpm.
6 boxes	50 bpm.

If the rate is slow or rhythm is irregular, count the number of QRS complexes between 2 three second slash marks at the top of the page (30 big boxes). Multiply the number of QRS complexes by ten to get the heart rate.

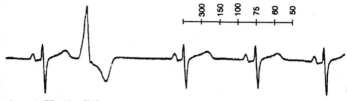

sinus rate 75, with a PVC

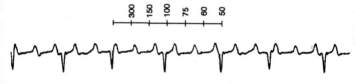

atrial rate 250, ventricular rate 100: atrial flutter with AV block

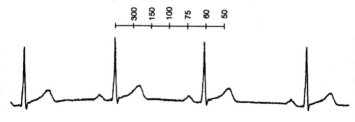

sinus rate 60

7

Rhythm

Questions for every rhythm:

1. What is the rate of the QRS?   Rate > 100 is called tachycardia.
    Rate < 60 is called bradycardia.

2. Is the QRS regular or irregular?   Irregular: Atrial fibrillation, extra
    beats superimposed on sinus,
    sinus arrhythmia, others.

3. Is the QRS narrow or wide?   A wide QRS indicates an
    impulse arises in the ventricle
    or conduction delay.

4. Are there P waves?   Look at the rhythm strip in more
    than one lead. Check leads II,
    V1 and V2.

5. Does a P wave precede every QRS?

6. Is the PR interval constant?

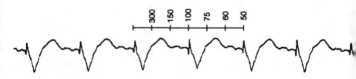

P waves, pacer spike, regular, wide complex, rate 100: atrial sensed and ventricular paced rhythm.

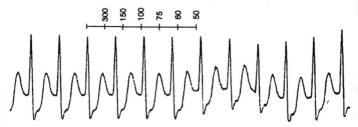

P waves not seen, regular, narrow, rate 190: SVT.

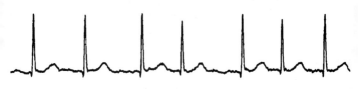

P waves not seen, irregular, rate 115: atrial fibrillation.

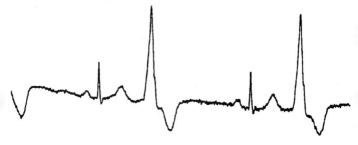

P wave seen with every other QRS, alternating narrow and wide QRS, rate 66: bigeminy.

Axis

The net amplitude of the QRS for any given lead indicates the net
electrical forces of the depolarizing heart in that particular direction.
Using multiple limb leads we can produce a two dimensional electrical
picture of the heart. The vector sum of any two limb leads yields the
axis.

At a minimum, memorize:

Lead I = 0°
Lead aVF = + 90°

Figure out which quadrant the axis is in by using leads I and aVF. By
convention the frontal plane is oriented so that the 0° is to the patient's
left, perpendicular to the long axis of the body.

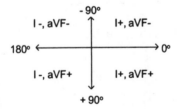

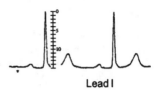

Lead I

Here, lead I is positive and lead aVF is negative, so the axis lies between 0° and -90°. Because lead I is so much larger than lead aVF, the axis would be closer to 0° than to -90°.

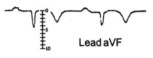

Lead aVF

Axis

Look for an isoelectric QRS, (a QRS where the deflection upward is equal to the deflection downward). The axis lies upon a line perpendicular to the isoelectric.

Thus, for any given isoelectric there are two perpendicular axes, an axis + 90° from the isoelectric and an axis - 90° from the isoelectric. The correct perpendicular axis lies in the quadrant determined by I and aVF.

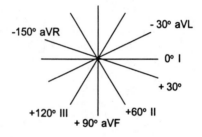

Positive QRS ← I

II

aVR

Isoelectric QRS ← III
+III

aVL

aVF

Positive QRS ←

Lead I is positive.
Lead aVF is positive.
The axis is between 0° and 90°.

Lead III is isoelectric.
(Lead III = +120°.)

There are two axes which are
perpendicular to lead III:
30° and 210° (-150°).

The axis is 30°.

PR Interval

The PR interval is measured from the beginning the P wave to the beginning of the QRS complex. The normal PR interval is less than 0.21 seconds.

Short PR:
An short PR interval, less than 0.12 seconds, is associated with the Wolf-Parkinson-White and Lown-Ganong-Levine syndromes. A short PR may also result from junctional or low atrial ectopic rhythms.

Long or dissociated PR:
   First degree AV block: a PR interval longer than 0.20 seconds.
   Second degree AV block: not every P wave results in a QRS.
      Type I or Wenckebach: PR interval progressively lengthens
         and eventually a QRS is dropped.
      Type II: the PR interval is constant, but P waves do not
         consistently lead to a QRS.
   Third degree AV block: also called complete heart block.
      P waves and QRS complexes are no longer related to each
      other. The atria and ventricles each move at their own regular
      rhythm. The ventricular (QRS) rate should be slower than the
      atrial (P wave) rate.

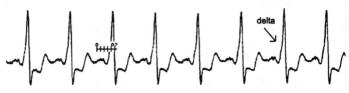

PR interval 0.10 seconds, delta wave (early upstroke of QRS): WPW.

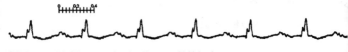

PR interval 0.25 seconds: 1st degree AV block.

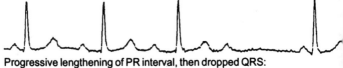

Progressive lengthening of PR interval, then dropped QRS:
2nd degree AV block, Mobitz I (Wenckebach).

QRS Interval

The QRS interval is measured from the start of the Q or R wave, whichever is first, to the end of S wave. The QRS is normally less than 0.12 seconds.

A lengthened QRS complex can result from three possibilities:

1. The beat initiated in the ventricle (i.e. PVC, VT, AIVR).

2. Impairment of the conduction system exists so that the wave of depolarization coming down from the atria does not or can not travel through all of the bundle branches (i.e. bundle branch block, aberrant ventricular conduction, WPW).

3. The ventricle is being paced.

QT interval

The QT interval is measured from the start of the QRS complex, to the end of the T wave.

Since the QT interval varies with the heart rate, the QT is "corrected" (denoted as QTc) to make comparisons between EKGs.

$$QTc = \frac{QT}{\sqrt{RR\ interval}}$$

The QTc interval equals the QT when the ventricular rate is 60 bpm, i.e. RR = 1 second. Normally, the QTc is less than 0.42 seconds in men, and less than 0.43 seconds in women. At normal sinus rates the QT should be equal to less than one half the length of the preceding RR interval.

Causes of a prolonged QT include:
    Antiarrhythmics, especially quinidine and procainamide.
    Other drugs such as phenothiazines and tricyclic antidepressants.
    Idiopathic (long QT syndrome).
    Hypothermia.
    Electrolyte abnormality.

P waves

Look for evidence of enlarged atria or abnormal conduction. The right atria is typically reflected in lead II and the left in lead V1.

Enlarged atria:
   Right Atrial Enlargement (RAE):
      Peaked P wave > 2.5 mm in lead II.

   Left Atrial Enlargement (LAE):
      Biphasic P wave in V1 with a 1 box wide and one box deep
      negative deflection. Double peaked P in lead II.

Abnormal conduction:
   In order to call a tracing sinus rhythm, the P wave must nearly
   always be upright in II, III and aVF. Inverted P waves in leads II,
   III, aVF imply a negative axis of the P wave or "retrograde"
   conduction in the atria due to a "low atrial" or junctional
   pacemaker.

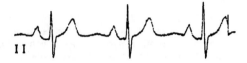

Peaked P wave in lead II, RAE.

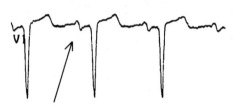

Biphasic P wave in lead V1, LAE.

Q waves

Q waves are the hallmark of infarction. Q waves generally occur after some degree of myocardial death, though some acute Qs are reversible with reperfusion.

If a Q wave is less than one box deep or one box wide, or is less than a third of the following R wave, it's significance may be questioned. The small Q is described as an embryonic, small, or nonsignificant Q. While most small Qs are benign, some will be associated with infarcted myocardium.

Infarction occurs in the territory of one or more coronary arteries. Typical infarction distributions are:

Territory	EKG leads	Artery
Anterior	V2-V6	LAD
Inferior	II, III, aVF	RCA
Lateral	I, aVL, V5, V6	Circumflex
Posterior	Tall R in V1-V2	Variable

The correlation of territory and coronary artery is an imprecise science in the age of angiogram.

Inferior Infarct Pattern

Rate - 60 beats per minute. Rhythm - sinus.
Intervals - PR = 0.16 seconds, QRS = 0.08 seconds, QT = 0.43 seconds.
Axis - leads I+ and aVF +, axis is >0° and <90°, isoelectric aVL, axis = 60°.
Normal P waves. Q waves in leads II, III, aVF. R wave early transition in V2.
Normal ST segments. Flattened T waves in lead III.
Interpretation: Inferior infarct; probably old.

R wave progression

The precordial leads are designed to measure electrical forces in the horizontal (i.e. precordial) plane. V1 and V2 pick up right ventricular and anterior left ventricular forces, while V5 and V6 pick up lateral ventricular forces.

In the normal EKG, R waves are small in V1-V2 and grow larger as one goes laterally. The R wave should be the dominant deflection in the QRS by V3 or V4. Interpreting R wave progression is performed with the knowledge that precordial R waves are very sensitive to lead placement.

Early R waves: R waves in leads V1 and V2 as large as those in the next several leads can reflect posterior infarction, lateral myocardial infarction, right ventricular hypertrophy or septal hypertrophy.

Poor R wave progression: R waves do not begin to dominate QRS until V5 or V6. This may represent infarction or injury of the anterior left ventricle and carries almost as much significance as Q waves.

R Wave Progression

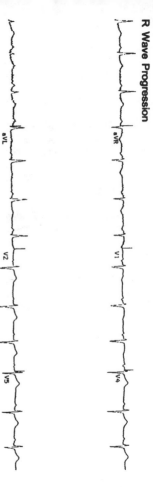

Rate - 65 beats per minute. Rhythm - sinus.
Intervals - PR = 0.16 seconds. QRS = 0.10 seconds. QT = 0.40 seconds.
Axis - leads I + and aVF -, axis is > -90° and < 0°, isoelectric close to aVF, axis = -10°.
Biphasic P wave in I. Q wave in aVF. Delayed R wave progression with transition in V5.
Normal ST segments and T waves.
Interpretation: LAE. Delayed R wave progression.

ST segments

The ST segment is the portion of the EKG between the end of the QRS and the beginning of the T wave. ST segments are examined for elevation or depression against the TP segment (not the PR intervals). The TP segment is the true isoelectric line. Never read ST changes from a monitor or a rhythm strip.

ST elevation is the hallmark of myocardial injury. The location of infarction is suggested by the leads in which ST segment elevation appears. Post MI, persistant elevations are associated with ventricular aneurysm. In young people, J-point elevation (concave up-sloping ST segments that take off a bit above isoelectric) is common and does not indicate pathology.

ST depression classically indicates ischemia. Remember that leads behind an area of injury may have ST depression that indicates injury. Likewise elevation may be depression seen from the opposite side of the heart.

Nonspecific ST-T changes, small or unclear elevation or depression, long flat ST segments suggest ischemia often until proven otherwise. Remember to check an old EKG. In a routine baseline study, they may mean nothing at all.

ST Segments

Rate - 70 beats per minute. Rhythm - sinus.

Intervals - PR = 0.18 seconds, QRS = 0.10 seconds, QT = 0.38 seconds.

Axis - leads I + and aVF +, axis is >0° and <90°, isoelectric aVL, axis = 60°.

Normal P waves. No Q waves. Early R wave with transition at V2.

ST sloping elevations V1-V4, largest is 3 mm J point elevation in lead V2. T waves upright except for aVR and aVL where they follow the complex.

Interpretation: Possible acute anterior injury.

T waves

T waves are observed for indications of ischemia or electrolyte disturbances. T waves are normally inverted in lead aVR, and normally upright in I, II, V3-V6. If the patient's old EKGs has abnormal T wave inversions which now are corrected, then some ischemia may be currently present and the T waves are said to be "pseudonormalized".

Flattened Ts may indicate ischemia.

Tall or "hyperacute" T waves are seen following MI. "Peaked" T waves (also known as T waves you would not want to sit on) are highly suggestive of hyperkalemia.

U waves

U waves are also associated with metabolic disturbances, typically hypokalemia and hypomagnesemia. They may be seen following the T wave. U waves make interpretation of the QT interval especially difficult.

T Wave Inversions

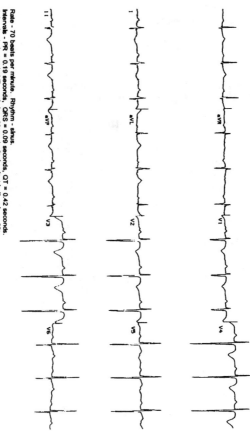

Rate - 70 beats per minute. Rhythm - sinus.
Intervals - PR = 0.19 seconds, QRS = 0.09 seconds, QT = 0.42 seconds.
Axis - leads I + and aVF -, axis is >-90° and <0°, isoelectric II, axis = -30°.
Normal P waves. No Q waves. R wave transition in V5.
ST segments isoelectric except for V5 minimally elevated.
T wave inversion in II, III, and aVF, as well as in V1 - V5.
Interpretation: Possible inferior and anterior ischemia.

Rhythm Disturbances

Extra Beats (i.e. Premature Beats or Extrasystoles)

Premature Atrial Contractions (PACs) occur when an ectopic atrial focus fires before the next anticipated sinus beat and results in a unusual looking P wave (often retrograde) and a normal (narrow) QRS. Frequently, the P wave is non-conducted because the beat falls very early on the refractory period of the AV node. In this case there will be a "dropped" QRS or ventricular pause that may be confused with bradycardia or heart block.

Premature Junction (Nodal) Beats occur when an ectopic beat arises in the AV junction before the next anticipated sinus beat. The QRS that follows is usually normal, and the P wave inscribed may precede, follow or be lost in the QRS. Because the atria are depolarizing retrograde, the P wave is usually inverted.

Premature Ventricular Contractions occur when an ectopic ventricular focus initiates a ventricular depolarization before a normal QRS is expected. Because the wave of ventricular depolarization is not initiated in the His-Purkinje system, it is slow causing a wide and sloppy QRS. A pause often follows from a blocked sinus excitation. There will be no preceding P wave for the PVC.

Abnormal Rhythms and Bradycardias

Rhythm	Rate	Morphology
Sinus bradycardia	<60	P waves (upright) seen.
Junctional bradycardia	40-60	Narrow QRS. P waves absent or dissociated and slower than the QRS.
Ventricular escape	30-40	Wide QRS. (Slow V-tach) P waves absent or dissociated.
Second Degree HB	20-60	Varying PR interval with dropped beat type I. Constant PR with dropped beat, type II.
Third Degree Heart Block	20-45	Lack of association P and QRS.
Normal Sinus Rhythm	60-100	Upright P wave, narrow QRS, normal intervals.
Accelerated Junctional	60-100	P waves retrograde, may precede, follow or be buried in QRS. Narrow, regular QRS.
Accelerated Idioventricular Rhythm (AIVR)	50-100	Wide complex QRS.
Atrial Fibrillation	50-200	Narrow, usually irregularly irregular QRS interval. No P waves seen.
Atrial Flutter	50-150	Narrow, regular QRS. No P waves but may have "saw tooth" character of atrial depolarization at 300 bpm.

Tachycardias

Rapid rhythms are first differentiated by whether the QRS inscribed is narrow (i.e. supraventricular) or wide. A wide QRS tachycardia is almost always ventricular tachycardia (VT) except when the supraventricular rhythm is being conducted "aberrantly."

Rhythm	Rate	Morphology
Sinus Tachycardia	100-160	P waves upright.
Paroxysmal Atrial Tachycardia	140-220	Regular. Abnormal P waves.
Multifocal Atrial Tachycardia	100-200	Three separate P wave morphologies.
Junction tachycardia	140-220	Regular. P wave may be hidden by QRS.
Ventricular tachycardia (VT)	150-250	Regular, wide QRS. P waves may or may not be seen, but are dissociated from the QRS.
Torsades de Pointes	200-250	VT with varying (undulating) amplitude of the QRS.
Ventricular fibrillation (VF)	>250	Chaotic. Look in more than one lead.

VT versus SVT with Aberrancy

Ventricular tachycardia is the more dangerous of the two. Lean towards considering wide complex tachycardias as VT particularly in the setting of coronary artery disease (until proven otherwise by EPS).

VT	SVT
QRS > 0.14 seconds.	QRS < 0.14 seconds.
Left Axis Deviation.	May be preceded by a PAC.
Constant Axis.	May respond to vagal maneuvers.
AV dissociation.	
Concordancy in V leads (same direction).	
Fusion and capture beats.	

30

Supraventricular Tachycardia

II

Rate - 180 beats per minute.   Rhythm - supraventricular tachycardia.
Intervals - PR = n/a, QRS = 0.08 seconds, QT = 0.12 seconds.
Axis - leads I and aVF +, axis is >0° and < +90°, isoelectric aVL, axis = + 60°.
P waves not seen. No Q waves.   R wave transition in V3 - V4.
ST globally depressed relative to PR segment - I, II, III, aVF, V1-V6. Elevated in aVR.
T waves upright, flat in III.
Interpretation: SVT.

Hypertrophy

Hypertrophied myocardium results in increased electrical forces and thus an increase in the magnitude of QRS deflection. Numerous morphological criteria have been developed. None are perfect.

Left Ventricular Hypertrophy

R in aVL > 11, or the sum of S in V1 and R in V5 or V6 >35 mm.
QRS duration >0.10 seconds.
Strain pattern with down-sloping ST segments, depression and asymmetric T wave inversion, V5-V6.
Left axis deviation in the absence of LBBB or left anterior fascicular block.
Left atrial enlargement.

Right Ventricular Hypertrophy

Right axis deviation >110 degrees in the absence of RBBB, posterior fascicular block or inferior MI or anterolateral MI.
Dominant R wave > 5 mm in V1.
R:S ratio >1.0 in V1.
RV strain pattern with ST segment depression and T wave inversion in V1-V3.

Left Ventricular Hypertrophy

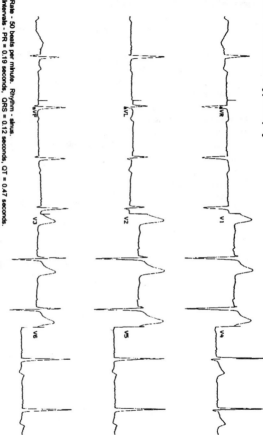

Rate - 50 beats per minute.   Rhythm - sinus.
Intervals - PR = 0.19 seconds.   QRS = 0.12 seconds.   QT = 0.47 seconds.
Axis - leads I + and aVF +, axis is > 0° and < 90°, closest to isoelectric aVL, axis = + 50°.
Small biphasic P waves in V1.   Relatively small Q waves II, III, and aVF.   R wave transition in V3.
R waves in V5 and V6 sum to 56 mm.
Normal ST segments.   Biphasic T waves in I, aVL, V5, V6.
Interpretation: LVH with strain.

Blocks - Left Bundle Branch Block

If the normal conducting system is damaged, one of two possibilities can result:

If the damage is at the site of the AV node or His bundle, conduction from atria to ventricle may be blocked. This is termed AV block and is manifest as heart block (i.e. 1st, 2nd, 3rd).
See pages 14-15.

If the damage is at the level of the bundle branches, i.e. infranodal, the ventricle will be stimulated inefficiently and a wide, sloppy QRS vector will result. Block of all three bundle branches can lead to complete heart block.

Left Bundle Branch Block (LBBB)

The wide QRS vector is directed leftward and posteriorly. Interpretation of ischemia or infarction is dubious in most hands.

QRS > 0.12 seconds.

Broad or notched R wave in the lateral precordial leads, I & aVL.

Q waves and S waves are usually absent.

Left axis deviation < 30°.

Left Bundle Branch Block (LBBB)

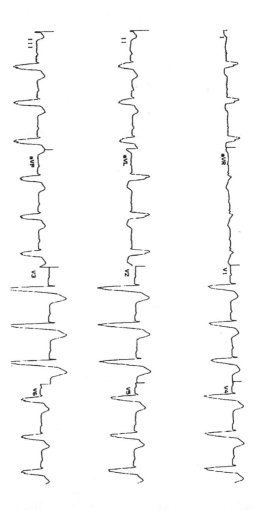

Rate - 80 beats per minute. Rhythm - sinus.
Intervals - PR = 0.20 seconds, QRS = 0.19 seconds, QT = 0.42 seconds.
Axis - leads I + and aVF -, axis is >-90° and <0°, isoelectric aVR, axis = -60°.
Normal P waves. Will not comment on Q waves, ST segments or T waves.
Interpretation: Left Bundle Branch Block and just shy of First Degree AV Block.

Right Bundle Branch Block (RBBB)

The terminal QRS vector directed rightward and anteriorly. Can read old MI by Q waves.

Large R in V1, large S in V4.

QRS >.12 seconds.

RSR' pattern in the anterior leads (V1-V3) with ST segment depression and T wave inversion.

Wide S wave in the lateral precordial leads (V5-V6) and lead I.

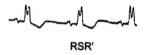

RSR'

note: an RSR' is not a mandatory finding.

Right Bundle Branch Block

Rate - 80 beats per minute. Rhythm - sinus.
Intervals - PR = 0.16 seconds, QRS = 0.14 seconds, QT = 0.40 seconds.
Axis - leads I + and aVF +, axis is > 0° and < 90°, isoelectric II, axis = + 30°.
Normal P waves. No Q waves. RSR' in V2.
Inverted T waves in V1 - V3.
Interpretation: Right Bundle Branch Block (RBBB).

Left Anterior Hemiblock

The inferior, posterior regions of the left ventricular endocardium are activated before the anterosuperior left ventricular area. The QRS duration is normal.

Left Axis from - 30° to -90° *

Small q wave in leads I and aVL.

R waves in II, III, aVF.

aVR shows a terminal positive deflection.

rS complexes are often seen in lead II with positive T waves.

* Right superior axis deviation is possible with either lateral myocardial infarction or right ventricular hypertrophy.

Left Anterior Hemiblock

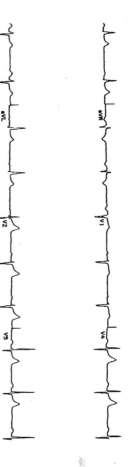

Rate - 60 beats per minute. Rhythm - sinus.
Intervals - PR = 0.19 seconds. QRS = 0.08 seconds. QT = 0.39 seconds.
Axis - leads I + and aVF - , axis is > -90° and < 0°, isoelectric aVR, axis = -60°.
Normal P waves. No Q waves.
Normal ST segments. RS in lead II with an upright T wave.
Interpretation: Left Anterior Fascicular Block.

Left Posterior Hemiblock

The impulse emerges from the unblocked anterosuperior division producing early depolarization changes as small inferior q waves. The spread of excitation rightward over the ventricle without the benefit of fascicles produces the evidence of right axis deviation.

Right axis, > 90°.

Small q waves in leads II, III, aVF.

Deep S waves in leads I and aVL.

R waves in leads II, III, and aVF.

Left Posterior Hemiblock

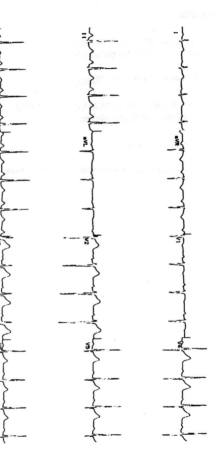

Rate - 88 beats per minute.   Rhythm - sinus.
Intervals - PR = 0.15 seconds. QRS = 0.10 seconds. QT = 0.36 seconds.
Axis - leads I + and aVF +, axis is > 0° and < 90°, close to isoelectric I, axis ≅ 90°.
Normal P waves. Small Q waves in III, III, and aVF. Normal R wave progression.
Normal ST segments. T waves follow QRS.
Interpretation: Left Posterior Hemiblock.

Pericarditis

Concave ST segment elevations diffusely,
especially in the precordial leads.

PR segment depression diffusely.

Evidence for effusion (think about tamponade)
Low voltage QRS complexes.

Electrical alternans.

In the later stages, T wave inversions are diffuse.

Cor Pulmonale

Pulmonary hypertension due to lung disease with secondary right ventricular hypertrophy. EKG relfects increased right ventricular voltages.

S1, Q3 pattern

Right axis deviation > 100 degrees.

S1, S2, S3 pattern.

R/S ratio in V6 is less than 1.0.

Pulmonary Embolus

Patients with significant pulmonary emboli usually have abnormal EKGs and commonly have findings of sinus tachycardia and nonspecific ST and T changes. The classic, rarely seen, findings in pulmonary embolus are described as "S1-QIII-TIII".

Other potential findings are:
Deep S wave in lead I.

Q wave in lead III.

Inverted T wave in lead III.

Right axis deviation.

Incomplete or complete RBBB.

All the abnormal rhythms associated with cardiac arrest.

Electrolyte and Drug Findings

Hyperkalemia

Sequential EKG manifestations as K+ rises above 6 mEq/L
include:

> Tall, peaked T waves.
> Depressed ST segments.
> Decreased amplitude of R waves.
> Prolongation of PR interval.
> Diminished to absent P waves.
> Widening of QRS.
> Widening of QT interval with sine wave pattern QRS
>   (Torsades de Pointes).
> Asystole.

Hyperkalemia
Hypokalemia

> T wave flattening.
> U waves.
> ST segment depression.

Hypercalcemia

> Decreased ST segments.
> Shortens QT interval.
> Tachycardia.

Hypocalcemia

> Prolonged QTc.

Electrolyte and Drug Findings (continued)

Digoxin
Sloped ST segment depression.
Atrial tachycardia.
AV block.
Accelerated junctional rhythms.
Ventricular tachycardia and fibrillation.

Beta-blockers
Sinus bradycardia.
AV block.

Calcium Channel Blockers
Sinus arrest.
AV block.

Quinidine/Procainamide/Disopyramide
QT prolongation.
Torsade de Pointes.

Amiodarone
Bradycardia.
Complete heart block.
QT prolongation.

Notes

Index

Order Form

	price	# ordered
The Intern Pocket Survival Guide Masterson	$6.00	_____
The CCU Intern Pocket Survival Guide Masterson/Rothenhaus	$6.00	_____
The ER Intern Pocket Survival Guide Rothenhaus/Masterson	$6.00	_____
The ICU Intern Pocket Survival Guide Masterson/Rothenhaus/Tenner	$6.00	_____
The Surgical Intern Pocket Survival Guide Chamberlain	$6.00	_____
The Intern Pocket Admission Book (contain blank admission forms)	$4.00	_____
The Pocket Guide to Eponyms and Subtle Signs of Disease Tenner/Masterson	$6.00	_____
The Housestaff Book of Forms (full size forms)	$7.50	_____
The EKG Pocket Survival Guide Masterson/Handler/Tenner/Rothenhaus	$6.00	_____
The Oncology Intern Pocket Survival Guide Tenner/Masterson/Rollhauser	$6.00	_____
Forthcoming - 1/15/94 Clinician's Handbook of Preventive Services, Part I, Children and Adolescents Office of Disease Prevention, Editor - Kamerow	$12.95	_____
Clinician's Handbook of Preventive Services, Part II, Adults Office of Disease Prevention, Editor - Kamerow	$12.95	_____
	subtotal	$_____

Name:

Address: P & H $ 0.75:

Phone: Total $_____

Send a check for your order to:
International Medical Publishing
3017 Wisteria Drive, #313, Germantown Maryland 20878